The ECG~

What does it tell?

J. Gardiner, SRN, RNT, RCNT, Cert. Ed (FE)
Nurse Teacher, Gloucestershire College of Nursing and Midwifery

Stanley Thornes (Publishers) Ltd

The ECG~
What does it tell?

First published in 1981 by Stanley Thornes (Publishers) Ltd
Old Station Drive, Leckhampton
CHELTENHAM, Glos. GL53 0DN

Reprinted 1983 with minor alterations
Reprinted 1984
Reprinted 1986
Reprinted 1987
Reprinted 1989 with updated information
Reprinted 1991

British Library Cataloguing in Publication Data

Gardiner, James
    The E.C.G.—what does it tell?
    1. Electrocardiography
    2. Cardiovascular disease nursing
    I. Title
    616.1'207'547   RC583.5.E5

    ISBN 0-85950-302-X

Produced by C.G.S. Studios, Cheltenham.
Printed in Great Britain at The Bath Press, Avon.

Contents

Preface

This book is intended for use by all personnel involved in the care and observation of the patient with a dysrhythmia; for both the advanced trained ambulance personnel involved in pre-hospital care, and also the nurses and junior medical staff who are involved in the in-hospital phase of patient care.

My thanks go to the advanced trained personnel of Gloucestershire Ambulance Service and to the staff of Cheltenham General Hospital who helped in the assessment and writing of this book.

1981   J. GARDINER
                                                            Gloucester

Also by the same author and publishers:

Cardiac Arrest – What do you do?

Introduction: What is an ECG?

An electrocardiogram (ECG) is a recording of the electrical activity of the heart, throughout the cardiac cycle (both normal and abnormal). The activity is usually picked up by electrodes placed on the patient's skin. The resultant electrocardiogram is amplified and may be displayed either on an oscilloscope screen or on paper. The electrodes on the skin pick up a wave of activity or *depolarization* moving along each cell, within the heart. This wave of depolarization causes contraction of the affected part. After contraction the muscle cell returns to its resting state, in other words it *repolarizes*. This activity may also be picked up by the skin electrodes. If the wave of depolarization moves towards the electrode it will result in a positive or upward deflection on the ECG. If the wave of depolarization moves away from the electrode the result is a negative or downward deflection of the ECG.

If the position of the electrode receiving the electrical impulses is varied the resultant deflections on the ECG may vary in pattern (figure 1).

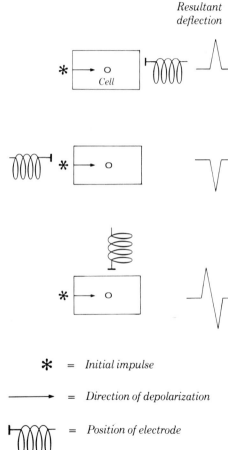

Figure 1 — The effect of depolarization on the ECG.

Resultant deflection

✱ = Initial impulse

⟶ = Direction of depolarization

⊦〰 = Position of electrode

The heart

The heart is a muscular pump which pumps deoxygenated blood from the body to the lungs, and oxygenated blood, from the lungs to the body. For this action to take place the heart is made up of two completely separate halves, each half consisting of a receiving chamber (*atrium*) and a pumping chamber (*ventricle*). There is a valve which prevents the back flow of the blood at the exit of each chamber. The muscle (*myocardium*) in the walls of each chamber is thinnest in the atria, which only have to pump blood into the ventricles, thicker in the right ventricle, which pumps the blood into the lungs, and thickest in the left ventricle which pumps the blood throughout the body. Within the myocardium is the *endocardium*, a smooth inner lining, and outside is the tough protective *pericardium* (figure 2).

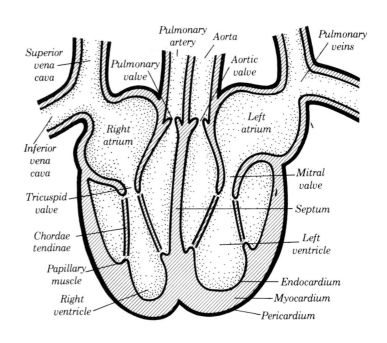

Figure 2. The heart

The conduction pathway

All cells within the heart can originate their own electrical activity which is then transmitted along a conduction 'pathway' of specialized cells (figure 3). The pathway consists of: the *sinoatrial (S-A) node*, a collection of cells situated in the wall of the right atrium near the entrance of the superior vena cava. Here depolarization is initiated at a rate of approximately 80 beats per minute.

The rate may be affected by the autonomic nervous system (the parasympathetic slows the rate and the sympathetic increases the rate), and also by the effect of some hormones. The impulse from the S-A node spreads across the atria causing a wave of

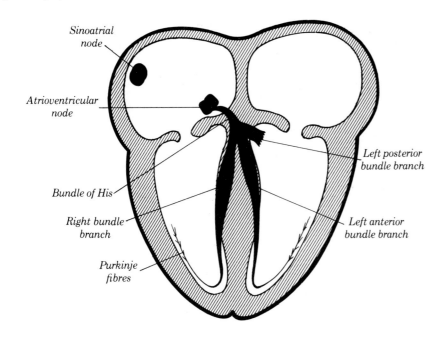

Figure 3. The electrical conduction pathway of the heart

Sinoatrial node

Atrioventricular node

Bundle of His

Right bundle branch

Purkinje fibres

Left posterior bundle branch

Left anterior bundle branch

depolarization which results in atrial contraction. The impulses then reach and pause at the *atrioventricular (A-V) node*. This is also a collection of specialized cells situated just to the right of the interatrial septum (near the coronary sinus).

After a slight pause the impulse is allowed to pass on. If for some reason the S-A node is unable to initiate any impulses the A-V node may do this but at a slower rate of approximately 60 beats per minute (normally the faster rate from the S-A node controls the

heart). Running from the A-V node into the posterior part of the interventricular septum is the electrical connection between the atria and the ventricles: *the bundle of His*. This is approximately 22 mm long and divides into its right bundle branch (to the right ventricle), and a much thicker left bundle branch. The latter divides almost immediately into an anterior branch (supplying the anterior part of the septum and left ventricle) and a posterior branch (supplying the posterior part of the septum and the posterior and inferior parts of the left ventricle).

Both branches end as numerous fine fibres running into the ventricular myocardium, known as *Purkinje fibres*. The impulse passed on from the A-V node passes very quickly along the bundle of His, bundle branches and Purkinje fibres, resulting in ventricular depolarization and contraction. In some circumstances impulses may originate in the Purkinje fibres (although at a rate of only 40 beats per minute or less). During ventricular depolarization the atria repolarize (that is, return to the previous resting state), after their depolarization the ventricles repolarize before the cycle starts again.

The normal ECG waveform

The normal waveform seen may vary depending upon the exact location of the skin electrodes. There are twelve different views normally used for diagnostic purposes — the twelve-lead ECG.

But for monitoring purposes, basically one of three leads or views are used — leads I, II or VI — which are positive leads, that is, the waveforms are mainly above the isoelectric line. All descriptions given are of the rhythm seen on lead I (figure 4).

The various waves seen on the ECG are labelled with letters to aid description — P, Q, R, S, T, U.

The first wave seen is the *P wave*. This is normally a positive (upright) deflection and is caused by atrial depolarization. After a slight pause the next three waves (Q, R, S) appear very close to each other and together represent ventricular depolarization. Often the waves are all present, but even if they are not (and this may be quite normal) the complex is known as a *QRS complex*.

The *Q wave* is often not seen at all and

Figure 4. The progress of depolarization (ECG leads I or II)

(a)

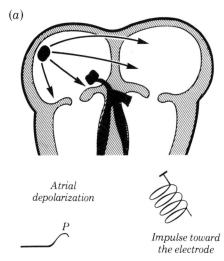

Atrial depolarization

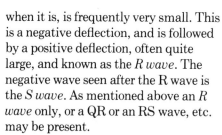

Impulse toward the electrode

(b)

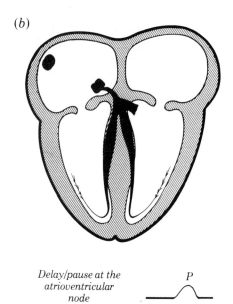

Delay/pause at the atrioventricular node

when it is, is frequently very small. This is a negative deflection, and is followed by a positive deflection, often quite large, and known as the *R wave*. The negative wave seen after the R wave is the *S wave*. As mentioned above an *R wave* only, or a QR or an RS wave, etc. may be present.

After a pause the QRS complex is followed by another positive wave, the *T wave* representing ventricular repolarization. Occasionally another

small positive wave may be seen after the T wave, known as the *U wave*. There are many differences of opinion over what exactly is the significance of the U wave. When seen on a single monitoring lead it must be correctly observed as a U wave and not an extra P wave (in fact, when seen the U wave is usually quite different from the P wave).

The pause between the P wave and the QRS complex (the pause of the impulse

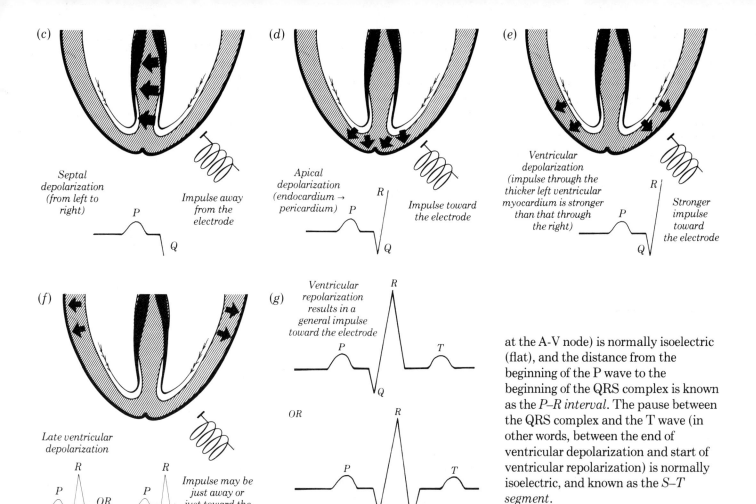

(c) Septal depolarization (from left to right)

Impulse away from the electrode

(d) Apical depolarization (endocardium → pericardium)

Impulse toward the electrode

(e) Ventricular depolarization (impulse through the thicker left ventricular myocardium is stronger than that through the right)

Stronger impulse toward the electrode

(f) Late ventricular depolarization

OR

Impulse may be just away or just toward the electrode

(g) Ventricular repolarization results in a general impulse toward the electrode

OR

at the A-V node) is normally isoelectric (flat), and the distance from the beginning of the P wave to the beginning of the QRS complex is known as the *P–R interval*. The pause between the QRS complex and the T wave (in other words, between the end of ventricular depolarization and start of ventricular repolarization) is normally isoelectric, and known as the *S–T segment*.

5

Timing

The ECG seen on the oscilloscope (monitor) and on paper can be recorded at various rates, although normally the rate of the paper is 25 mm/sec.
There are both vertical and horizontal lines on the paper. The horizontal lines indicate voltage of the waveform and are normally standardized at 10 mm (two large squares) equalling 1 millivolt (mV). The vertical lines indicate time, at a rate of 25 mm/sec, each large square (5 mm) is equal to 0.2 sec, and each small square (1 mm) is equal to 0.04 sec. These can be used in the estimation of intervals in the ECG and the atrial and/or ventricular rate (figure 5).

Figure 5(a). Normal ranges of intervals on the ECG

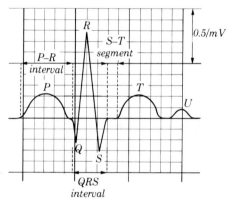

P–R interval adult — 0.18–0.2 sec
child — 0.15–0.18 sec

QRS interval — 0.07–0.1 sec

Figure 5(b). Calculation of rate

(Only accurate if the rhythm is regular.) (i) Count the number of QRS complexes in a three second period (15 large squares) and multiply by 20.

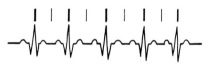

(ii) Find an R wave (or similar obvious wave, such as S) on a thick vertical line; divide the number of large squares between that R wave and the same wave on the next complex into 300. For example, (above)

$$\frac{300}{2} = 150 \; bpm.$$

(iii) As (ii) but divide the number of small squares between complexes into 1500. For example,

$$\frac{1500}{10} = 150 \; bpm.$$

Sinus rhythm

Description

Normal rhythm, with the impulse originating in the sinoatrial node, and following a normal pathway (figure 6).

ECG characteristic

- Rate: 60–100 bpm
- Rhythm: regular
- P waves: normal, preceding each QRS complex
- P–R interval: normal (0.16–0.2 sec)
- QRS complex: normal

Clinical significance

Nil, as this is a normal rhythm, therefore no treatment is required.

Figure 6. Sinus Rhythm

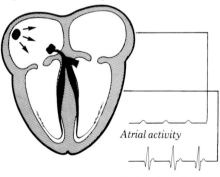

Atrial activity

Ventricular activity

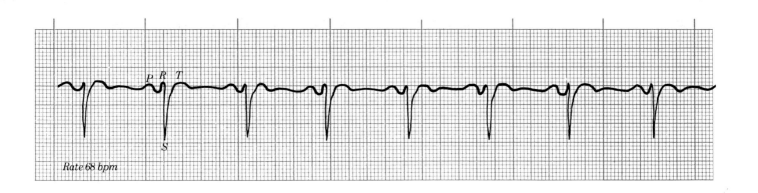

P R T

S

Rate 68 bpm

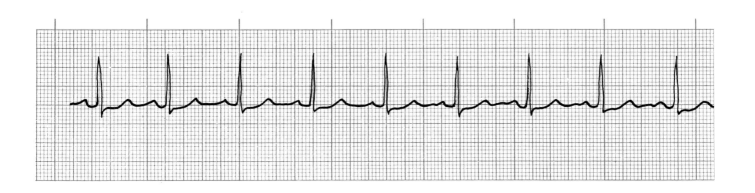

Sinus dysrhythmias

Sinus bradycardia

Description
Impulse originates in the sinoatrial node (figure 7).

ECG characteristic
- Rate: below 60 bpm (usually 40–60)
- Rhythm: regular
- P waves: normal
- P–R interval: normal
- QRS complex: normal

Clinical significance
May be normal in athletic young adults, or due to increased parasympathetic tone (vagus nerve), damage to S-A node, hypoxia or excess of cardiac drugs (such as *digoxin, propranolol*).
The slow rate may result in a lowering of the blood pressure and deterioration in tissue perfusion.

Treatment
No treatment is required if the blood pressure is maintained and the patient is unaffected generally. However, treatment may be required if:
(1) Blood pressure is unduly lowered (systolic < 100 mm Hg).
(2) Skin is pale, cold and clammy.
(3) There is agitation, confusion, dizziness or unconsciousness.
(4) Ventricular arrhythmias appear.
The drug of choice is *atropine sulphate* [600 mcg (0.6 mg) in 1 ml] in a dose of 0.6–1.2 mg i.v. to increase the heart rate.
The patient should also be placed flat to assist cerebral supply, and oxygen therapy given to reduce the risk of cerebral hypoxia (which may be causing the bradycardia).

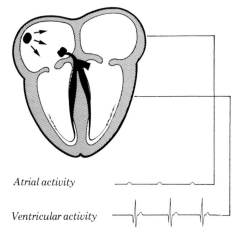

Figure 7. Sinus bradycardia

Atrial activity

Ventricular activity

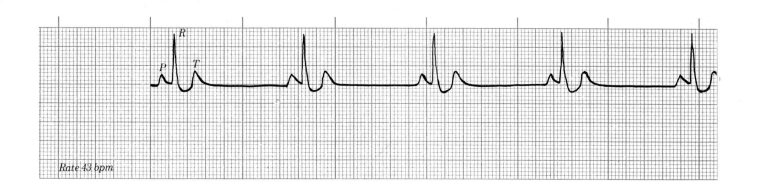

Rate 43 bpm

P R T

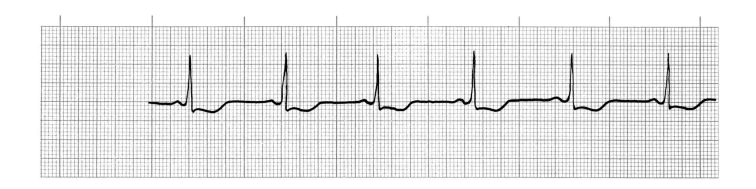

Sinus tachycardia

Description
Impulse originates in the sinoatrial node (figure 8).

ECG characteristic
- Rate: 100–180 bpm
- Rhythm: regular
- P waves: normal; if the rate is very fast the P wave may be buried in the T wave of the previous beat
- P–R interval: normal
- QRS complex: normal

Clinical significance
May be due to increased sympathetic stimulation caused by pain, fever or anxiety, or may be the normal reaction to exercise. It may also be due to haemorrhage, early hypoxia, congestive cardiac failure, left ventricular failure, or overdose of drugs such as *atropine, adrenaline, isoprenaline* or *aminophylline.*

If the rate is not too high there may be little effect on the patient. If over 120–140 bpm the cardiac output may be reduced due to decreased ventricular filling time. This may result in a lowered blood pressure, reduced tissue perfusion and its associated signs and symptoms.

The increased cardiac workload, but decreased coronary supply to the myocardium, may result in myocardial ischaemia and the possibility of chest pain.

Treatment
Relieve pain if present by *entonox* or other analgesia; reassure the patient; relieve anxiety (with *Valium* if necessary); relieve hypoxia with oxygen therapy; control haemorrhage; treat heart failure, if present, by *digoxin* and diuretics.

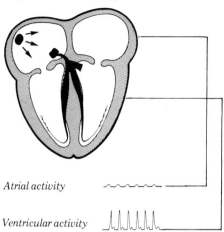

Figure 8. Sinus tachycardia

Atrial activity

Ventricular activity

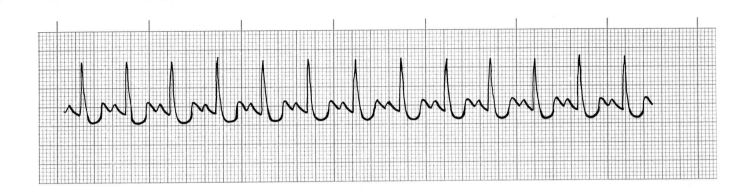

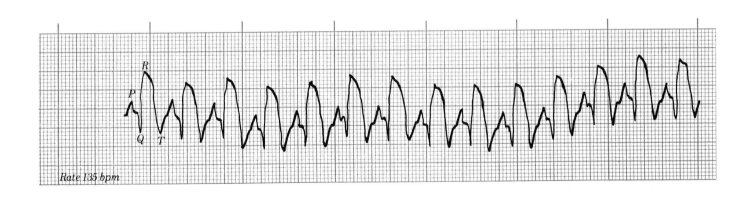

Rate 135 bpm

Sinus arrhythmia

Description
Impulse originates in the sinoatrial node, but the rate at which the impulses appear varies. If the patient's respiratory rate is observed, note that the heart rate increases during inspiration and decreases during expiration (figure 9).

ECG characteristic
- Rate: variable (but normally between 60–100 bpm)
- Rhythm: irregular (but regularly irregular in relation to respiration)
- P waves: normal
- P–R interval: normal
- QRS complex: normal

Clinical significance
This is accepted as a normal phenomenon in young people, when caused by variations in the parasympathetic activity on the sinoatrial node during respiration. An uncommon form of sinus arrhythmia which occurs without any apparent relationship to respiration or external factors may be indicative of heart disease.

Treatment
As this is a normal phenomenon no treatment is required.

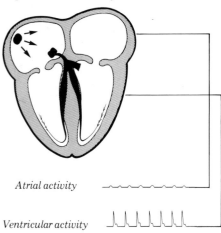

Figure 9. Sinus arrhythmia

Atrial activity

Ventricular activity

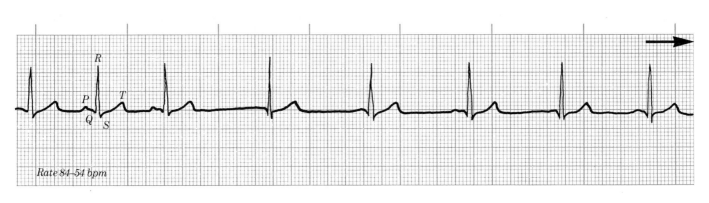

Rate 84–54 bpm

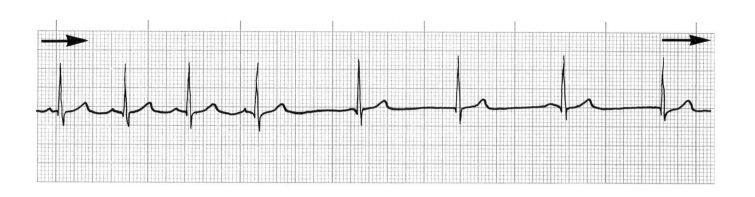

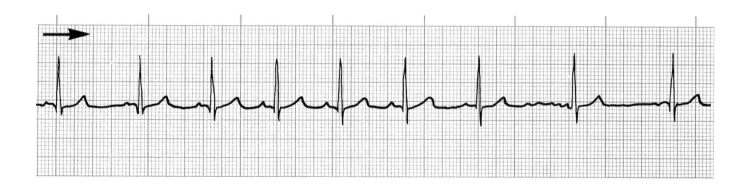

13

Sinus arrest

Description

The impulse originates in the sinoatrial node, resulting in a sinus rhythm or sinus bradycardia. But there is a pause in the rhythm due to a failure of the S-A node to originate an impulse, and this results in a completely missed beat, following which the previous rhythm may be recommenced. There may be other periods of sinus arrest (figure 10). The distance between the R wave prior to the sinus arrest and the R wave after, may or may not be double the normal R–R interval.

Occasionally another ectopic focus in the heart (atria, A-V node or ventricles) may appear during the pause as an escape beat. Note that the distance between the R wave prior to the sinus arrest and the R wave of the escape beat is greater than the normal R–R interval. The P wave of the escape beat (if present) may be abnormal, the QRS complex may or may not be normal depending upon the origin of the escape beat. The R–R interval from the escape beat to the next normal beat may be normal or slightly greater than normal.

ECG characteristic

- Rate: normal (60–100 bpm) or slow
- Rhythm: normal except for the pause left by the missed beat
- P waves: absent during sinus arrest otherwise normal (may be abnormal or absent if escape beat is present)
- P–R interval: absent during sinus arrest, otherwise normal
- QRS complex: absent during sinus arrest, otherwise normal (may or may not be normal if escape beat is present)

Clinical significance

If rate is otherwise normal the patient will be unaffected. The cause may be increased parasympathetic activity, or it may be drug-induced (such as through an excess of digoxin) or appear as a result of ischaemic heart disease. If the overall heart rate is low (<50 bpm) the patient may suffer the effects of a lowered cardiac output, and will need to be treated to relieve the symptoms of the lowered cardiac output (see sinus bradycardia). If caused by digoxin excess the drug may be withheld until the blood level is lower.

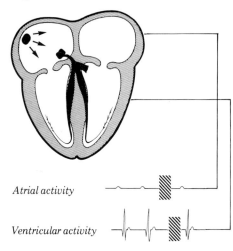

Figure 10. Sinus arrest

Atrial activity

Ventricular activity

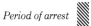

Period of arrest

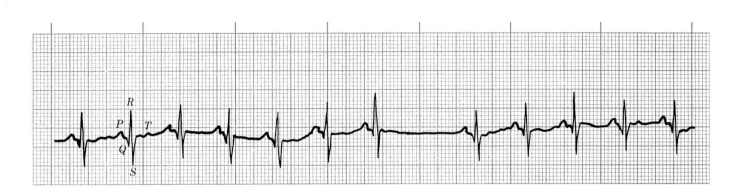

15

Supra-ventricular dysrhythmias

Wandering atrial pacemaker

Description
The impulses may originate in the S-A node, anywhere in the atria or in the A-V node. The site of impulse continually changes, resulting in varying shapes and sizes of the P wave, the QRS will remain normal (figure 11).

ECG characteristic
- Rate: normal
- Rhythm: slightly irregular (may appear regular)
- P waves: vary in size and shape depending on the exact origin of the impulse
- P–R interval: varies depending upon site of impulse (from 0.2 sec at the S-A node to 0.12 sec at the A-V node)
- QRS complex: normal

Clinical significance
May be a relatively normal phenomenon caused by increased parasympathetic stimulation, excessive digoxin, or ischaemic heart disease. It does not usually affect the patient, although it may be a warning of other atrial dysrhythmias.

Treatment
If the rhythm has no effect on the patient then no treatment is required, although the digoxin therapy may need to be altered if this is the cause of the dysrhythmia.

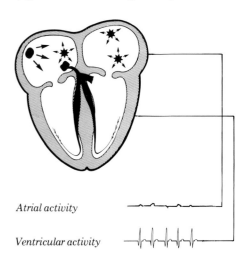

Figure 11. Wandering atrial pacemaker

Atrial activity

Ventricular activity

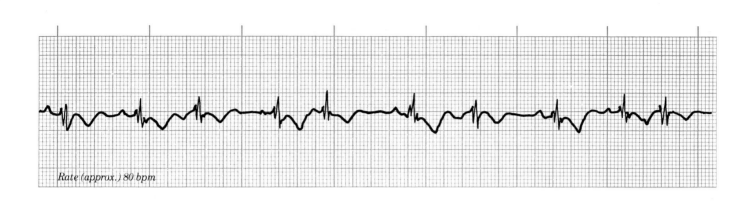

Rate (approx.) 80 bpm

Premature atrial contractions (atrial ectopics)

Description
A premature beat arises from an ectopic focus which originates an impulse before the next normal beat is due. Therefore in an otherwise 'normal' rhythm an ectopic beat appears. The R–R interval between the ectopic beat and the previous normal beat will be less than the normal R–R interval. The R–R interval between the ectopic beat and the following normal beat may be longer than the normal R–R interval. The pause after the ectopic beat, and before the next normal beat, is known as a *compensatory pause*. After the atrial ectopic the rhythm returns to normal until the next ectopic beat (figure 12).

ECG characteristic
- Rate: normal
- Rhythm: basically regular except for the atrial ectopics
- P waves: basically normal, but abnormal prior to the atrial ectopics
- P–R interval: normal, except that of the atrial ectopic and then will vary

depending upon the site of the ectopic focus.
- QRS complex: normal

Clinical significance
Premature atrial contractions may be a normal phenomenon and may be caused by emotional disturbances or the use of tobacco, tea or coffee. They may also be due to digoxin toxicity or to organic heart disease causing damage to the atrial wall. The presence of atrial ectopics (if very frequent) may be a warning of other atrial dysrhythmias.

Treatment
Usually no treatment required unless:
(1) The dysrhythmia is due to digoxin toxicity, assess blood level and alter the regime.
(2) The dysrhythmia is due to atrial damage/heart failure, in which case digoxin or other anti-dysrhythmics may be prescribed.

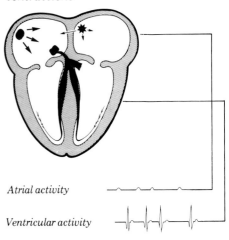

Figure 12. Premature atrial contractions

Atrial activity

Ventricular activity

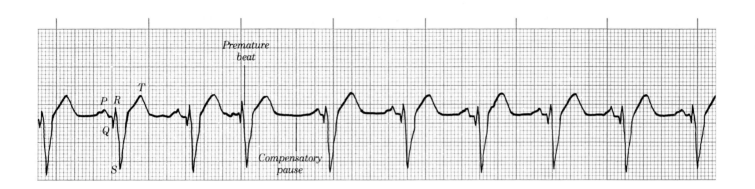

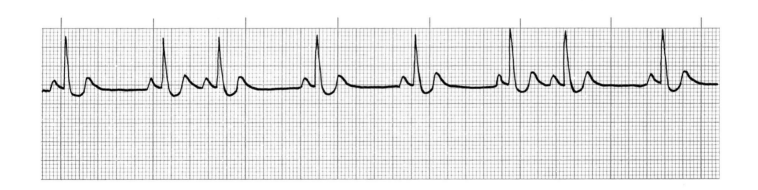

Atrial flutter

Description

The impulses originate within the atria. Either one or several ectopic foci initiate impulses very rapidly (at a rate of 220–350 times per minute). There is also a theory of a circular movement of impulses within the atria with the same effect. The rapid atrial rate gives rise to a sawtooth appearance on the ECG (known as F waves).

The ventricles are unable to respond to such a rapid rate, so the A-V node blocks many of the impulses resulting in more F waves than QRS complexes (figure 13).

ECG characteristics

- Rate: atrial rate 220–350/min. Ventricular rate varies with degree of block at the A-V node, which may be 60–180 bpm
- Rhythm: Atrial rhythm is regular. Ventricular rhythm often regular but may be irregular if the degree of block varies
- P waves: None seen — instead the characteristic sawtoothed flutter waves
- P–R interval: difficult to determine; F–R interval may be apparently normal on the complexes conducted through the A-V node
- QRS complex: normal

Clinical significance

If the ventricular rate is normal there may be little effect on the patient. If the ventricular rate is rapid, >140/min, there may be some loss in cardiac output, resulting in a lowered blood pressure, reduced tissue perfusion and associated signs and symptoms, due to reduced ventricular filling time. There may be some chest pain due to increased ventricular workload and decreased coronary artery flow (and therefore decreased oxygen supply to the myocardium).

The dysrhythmia may occur because of organic heart disease, damage to the atria, congestive cardiac failure or increased sympathetic tone. If due to disease, such as rheumatic heart disease or thyrotoxicosis, the arrhythmia may progress to atrial fibrillation.

Treatment

If the ventricular rate is normal the patient may be unaffected, but if it is rapid the patient may show the signs and symptoms of a lowered cardiac output.

Initially the treatment will be supportive — patient at rest (in position of the most comfort) — upright if dyspnoeic, flat if hypotensive. Oxygen therapy is given (or entonox if the patient complains of pain). The patient can then be treated with digoxin *or cardioversion* (synchronised DC shock), together with the treatment of any associated disease.

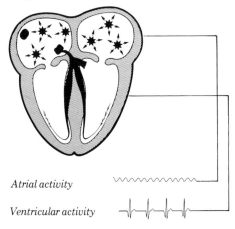

Figure 13. Atrial flutter

Atrial activity

Ventricular activity

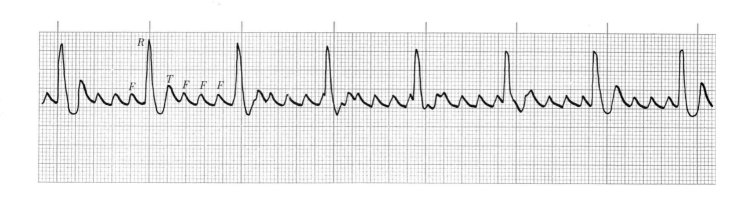

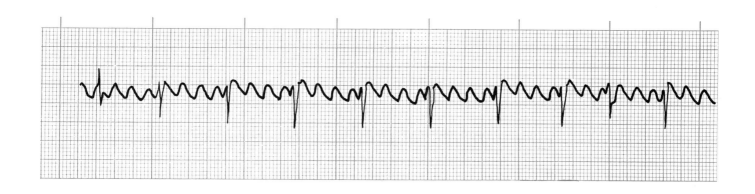

Atrial fibrillation

Description
Similar to that of atrial flutter, but there are usually more atrial ectopic foci and the atrial rate is in excess of 360 bpm, resulting in a completely uncoordinated twitching of the atria. There is a very variable rate of block at the A-V node resulting in a totally irregular response by the ventricular myocardium, so the ventricular rate is very irregular (irregularly irregular) and between 60–160 bpm. Because of the rate and irregularity some of the beats are poor in volume and may not be felt at the radial pulse (the difference in heart rate and radial pulse rate is known as the *pulse deficit*). The fibrillation waves seen on the ECG may vary in amplitude and may be either coarse or fine in appearance (figure 14).

ECG characteristic
- Rate: atrial rate >360/min; ventricular rate 60–160/min
- Rhythm: totally irregular
- P waves: none seen, only small irregular F waves
- P–R interval: not identifiable
- QRS complexes: normal

Clinical significance
May be due to increased sympathetic tone, damage to the atria due to organic heart disease, congestive cardiac failure, or associated with mitral valve disease.
If the ventricular rate is rapid there may be a lowering of cardiac output, as with atrial flutter.

Treatment
See atrial flutter (page 20)

Atrial flutter/ fibrillation

Occasionally the ECG will show a combination of atrial flutter and atrial fibrillation on the same trace. This may be termed a *flutter/fibrillation*.

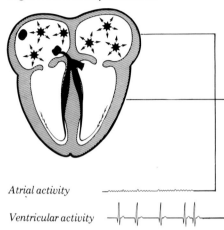

Figure 14. Atrial fibrillation

Atrial activity

Ventricular activity

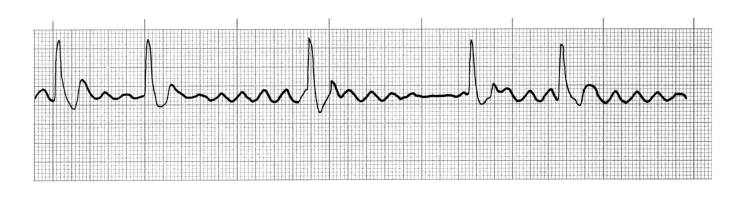

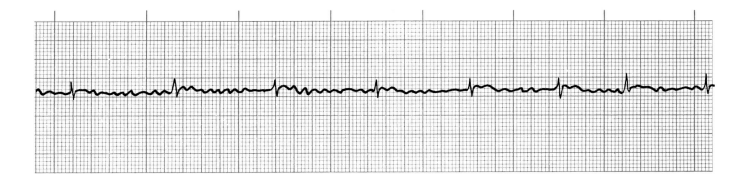

Junctional (nodal) rhythm

Description
If the impulse should originate from within the A-V node, either as an ectopic beat, escape beat or a complete rhythm, it is termed a junctional or nodal ectopic, beat or rhythm. The impulse originating in the region of the A-V node travels both up into the atria (retrograde conduction) and down into the ventricles.

If the S-A node does not function the A-V node may take over as the pacemaker of the heart. The ventricular rate then being approximately 40–65 bpm. The rhythm may be temporary or permanent, and the rate may increase up to 200 bpm if a tachycardia is present (figure 15).

There are three main areas from which the impulse may arise:
(1) Just above the A-V node (high nodal),
(2) Within the A-V node (mid-nodal), or
(3) Just below the A-V node (low nodal),
all resulting in a slight difference on the ECG.

High nodal
The impulse has time to activate the atria before the A-V node allows the impulse to pass on to the ventricles, so an inverted P wave is seen prior to the QRS complex.

Mid-nodal
The impulse reaches the atria at the same time as it reaches the ventricles, so no P wave is seen prior to the QRS complex, but a notch may be seen on it.

Low nodal
The impulse reaches the ventricles before the A-V node allows the impulse to pass on to the atria, so the P wave (inverted) is seen *after* the QRS complex but *before* the T wave.

All three types are generally classed together as junctional or nodal.

ECG characteristic
- Rate: normal 40–65/min (rarely up to 200/min)
- Rhythm: regular
- P waves: may be inverted prior to the complex, lost in the complex or inverted after the complex
- P–R interval: variable or absent
- QRS complex: normal but may be distorted if the P wave is buried in the complex (mid-nodal)

Clinical significance
The dysrhythmia may be due to damage to the A-V node in ischaemic heart disease, increased sympathetic activity (tachycardia), increased parasympathetic activity (bradycardia), congestive cardiac failure, hypoxia or overdosage of some cardiac drugs.

If the occasional nodal ectopic only is noted there are unlikely to be any ill-effects.

If there is a very slow or very fast ventricular rate there may be some loss of cardiac output, resulting in hypotension, reduced tissue perfusion (pale, cold, clammy skin) and, if a fast rate, chest pain.

Treatment
If there is no effect on the patient then no treatment is required.

If the dysrhythmia results in a lowering of cardiac output supportive treatment will be required (oxygen therapy, entonox, etc.). If the rate is slow atropine sulphate 600 mcg i.v., or *isoprenaline* by infusion may be effective, or a pacemaker insertion may be necessary.

If the rate is rapid vagal stimulation or the use of anti-dysrhythmics may be required (see supraventricular tachycardia page 28).

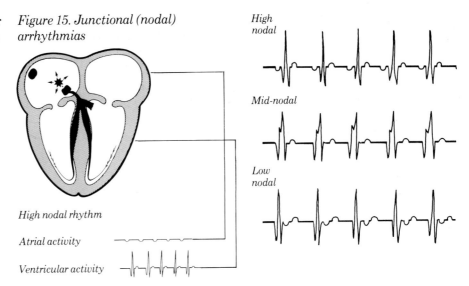

Figure 15. Junctional (nodal) arrhythmias

High nodal rhythm

Atrial activity

Ventricular activity

High nodal

Mid-nodal

Low nodal

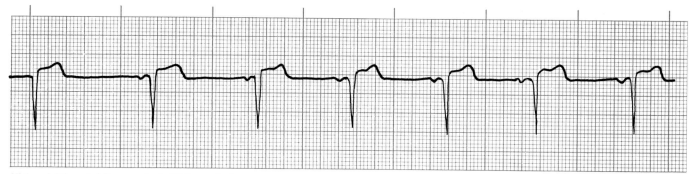

High nodal (inverted P wave prior to QRS complex)

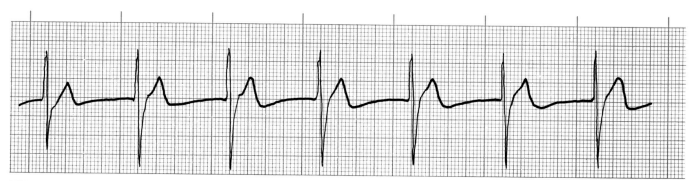

Mid-nodal (inverted P wave as a notch on the QRS complex)

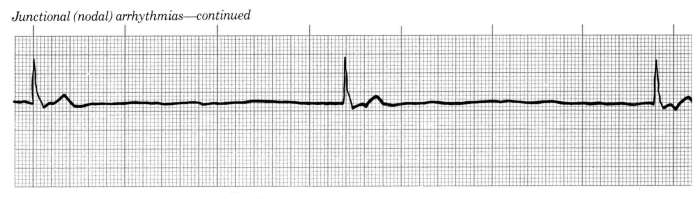

Low nodal (inverted P wave between QRS complex and T wave)

Paroxysmal atrial tachycardia

Very similar to supraventricular tachycardia, the difference being that the P waves are identifiable, so a more accurate identification than supraventricular tachycardia can be given. Both the effect and the treatment will be the same (if the rate is very rapid).

Supraventricular tachycardia

Description
The impulses originate from somewhere within the atria (including the S-A node and A-V node). Because of the rapid ventricular rate (>150/min) P waves cannot be identified so neither can the exact origin of the impulse. This term is therefore used as a blanket term when the rhythm originates above the ventricles (supraventricular) and because of the rapid rate it is difficult or impossible to identify the rhythm accurately (figure 16).
The arrhythmia may appear as paroxysms which start and end suddenly.

ECG characteristic
- Rate: 160–210/min (can reach 300/min in infants)
- Rhythm: regular
- P waves: cannot be identified
- P–R interval : cannot be identified
- QRS complex: normal, but occasionally an abnormality in the conduction of the impulse down the bundle branches (bundle branch block) may widen the QRS complex

and it may then be difficult to differentiate between supraventricular tachycardia and ventricular tachycardia.

Clinical significance
May occur for no apparent reason or may be due to damage to the S-A node, atria or A-V node (because of ischaemic heart disease). May also be caused by drug excess or sympathetic overactivity.
The very rapid rate will result in a lowering of cardiac output, with accompanying hypotension, poor tissue perfusion and cerebral hypoxia. The patient may complain of chest pain because the rapid rate may result in some myocardial ischaemia.

Treatment
Oxygen therapy or entonox may be required to treat the hypoxia and/or chest pain. Reflex vagal stimulation can be used (for example, carotid sinus massage or supraorbital pressure), in conjunction with monitoring of ECG and pulse, to reduce the rate; vera-pamil (Cordilox) 5 mg i.v. may be used (can be repeated, if necessary), or if unsuccessful other drugs such as digoxin, amiodarone or similar may be used, or elective cardioversion (especially if the cardiac output is very low).

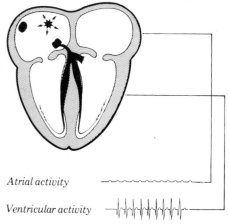

Figure 16. Supraventricular tachycardia

Atrial activity

Ventricular activity

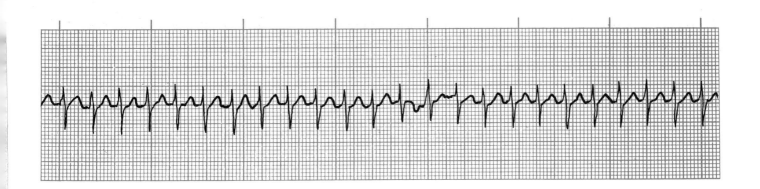

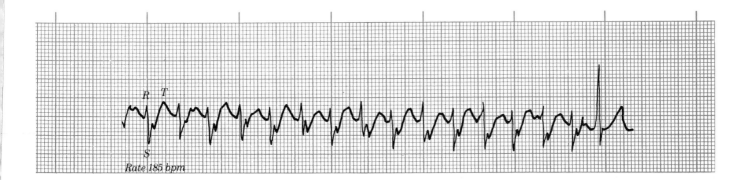

Rate 185 bpm

Ventricular dysrhythmias

Premature ventricular contractions (ventricular ectopics)

Description

The impulse originates somewhere within the ventricular myocardium. It is a premature beat arriving before the next normal beat is due and is followed by a compensatory pause. The QRS complex is wide and bizarre-looking (greater than 0.12 sec in duration) and the T wave is usually in the opposite direction to the QRS complex. The ectopic beat must just appear singly in an otherwise normal rhythm (figure 17).

ECG characteristic

- Rate: normal
- Rhythm: regular except for ventricular ectopics
- P waves: not seen
- P–R interval: not identifiable
- QRS complex: wide and bizarre (greater than 0.12 sec — three small squares).

Clinical significance

May be caused by damage to the ventricles (ischaemic heart disease), increased sympathetic or parasympathetic activity, hypoxia, acidosis, congestive cardiac failure or an overdose of some drugs.

Isolated ventricular ectopics may not be significant, but more frequent ventricular ectopics may result in a slight reduction in cardiac output, or may be the precursor of more serious ventricular dysrhythmias.

Treatment

May solely be observation (if the ectopics are associated with ischaemic heart disease), but if the ventricular ectopics are very frequent and/or lead to a lowering in cardiac output treat with *lignocaine* (see ventricular tachycardia page 34).

Figure 17. Premature ventricular contraction

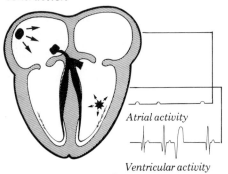

Atrial activity

Ventricular activity

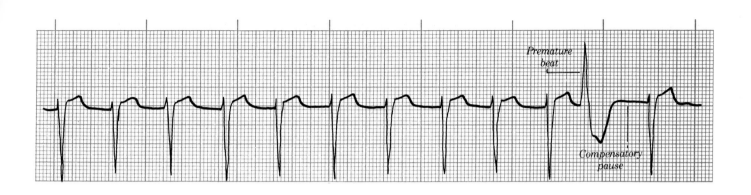

Premature beat

Compensatory pause

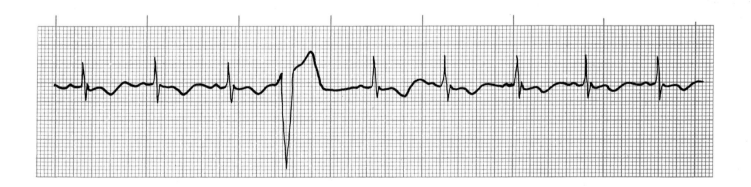

R-on-T ectopics

Description
The impulse originates somewhere in the ventricular myocardium, the same as ventricular ectopics (VEs). But with this type of VE the impulse is initiated earlier still so that the R wave of the VE lands on the T wave of the previous beat (in other words depolarization starts to occur while repolarization is still occurring) (figure 18).

ECG characteristic
- Rate: normal
- Rhythm: regular, except for the VEs
- P waves: not seen
- P–R interval: not identifiable
- QRS complex: wide and bizarre (greater than 0.12 sec), with the R wave of the VE apparently running off the T wave of the previous beat.

Clinical significance
The same as for VEs but with a greater risk of more serious ventricular dysrhythmias. Because depolarization starts again while repolarization is still occurring there is an increased risk of ventricular fibrillation.

Treatment
Close observation and drug therapy (lignocaine i.v.) as soon as possible (see ventricular tachycardia page 34).

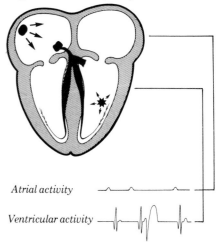

Figure 18. R-on-T ectopic

Atrial activity

Ventricular activity

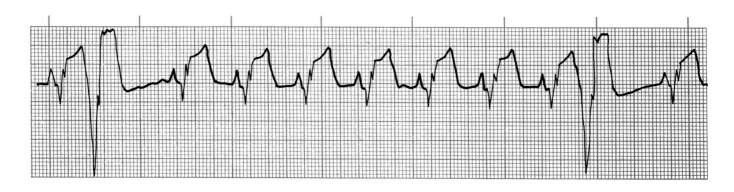

Ventricular bigeminy

In ventricular bigeminy every other beat is a ventricular ectopic, alternating with a normal beat. The interval between the normal beat and the ventricular ectopic is usually constant (figure 19).

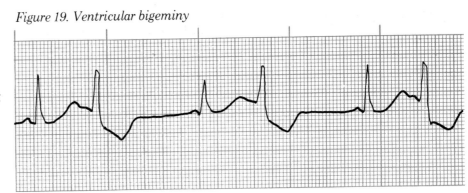

Figure 19. Ventricular bigeminy

Ventricular trigeminy

Either every third beat is a ventricular ectopic or each normal beat is followed by two ventricular ectopics (figure 20).

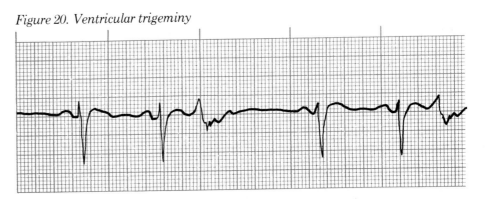

Figure 20. Ventricular trigeminy

Ventricular tachycardia

Description
Impulses originate from somewhere within the ventricular myocardium, appearing as three or more ventricular ectopics in a row. The ectopic foci may fire off at a rate of 140–220 bpm. It may sometimes be difficult to distinguish between ventricular tachycardia and supraventricular tachycardia, but note that ventricular tachycardia is slightly irregular while supraventricular tachycardia is regular (figure 21).

ECG characteristic
- Rate: usually 140–220 bpm
- Rhythm: slightly irregular
- P waves: usually present but may be buried in the QRS complex
- P–R interval: unidentifiable; the atria and ventricles are dissociated from each other
- QRS complex: wide and bizarre (greater than 0.12 sec)

Clinical significance
The rhythm may be caused by damage to the conduction pathway or ventricles (ischaemic heart disease), increased sympathetic or parasympathetic tone, hypoxia, acidosis, low serum potassium or overdose of some drugs.

If the rate is over 120–140 bpm the cardiac output may be significantly affected resulting in a drop in both tissue perfusion and blood pressure. The signs and symptoms noted would be those of poor tissue perfusion and hypotension, and the rapid heart rate may be associated with myocardial ischaemia (angina) and pump failure. The dysrhythmia itself can be extremely dangerous resulting in unconsciousness and even death. Ventricular tachycardia may be a precursor of ventricular fibrillation.

Treatment
If the patient is conscious, lignocaine is the drug of choice, given as: 2% lignocaine (100 mg in a prepacked 5 ml syringe) at a dose of 1mg/kg body weight i.v. (50–100 mg i.v. in the average adult). The dose may be repeated once more if necessary. Care must be taken when giving lignocaine i.v. because if given too quickly it may cause cerebral irritation resulting in a 'lignocaine fit'.

The i.v. dose should be followed by an intravenous infusion of 5% *dextrose with lignocaine* [5 ml of 20% lignocaine = 1000 mg, is added to 500 ml of 5% dextrose and run through a Metriset at 60 drops/min (60 ml/hour)].

If the patient loses consciousness because of an inadequate cardiac output, observe closely as he may lose his cardiac output completely in which case treat as cardiac arrest (see page 52).

Other antiarrhythmic drugs can be used such as disopyramide, flecainide or bretylium.

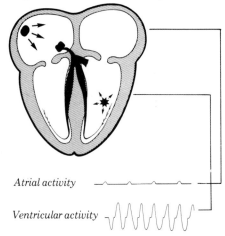

Figure 21. Ventricular tachycardia

Atrial activity

Ventricular activity

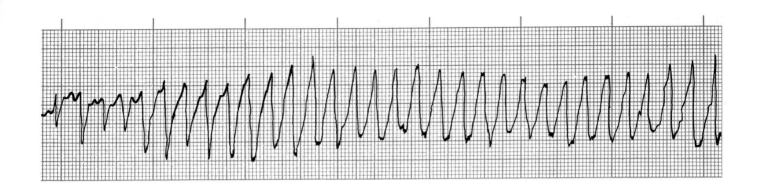

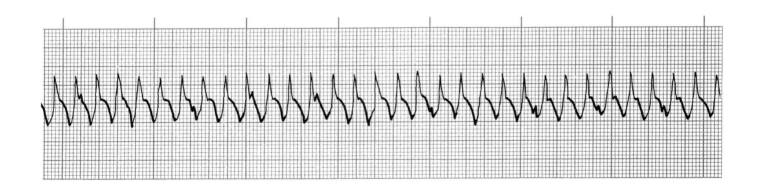

35

Ventricular fibrillation

Description
Impulses originate in one or more foci within the ventricles at a very fast rate, resulting in an uncoordinated activity within the ventricular myocardium (figure 22).

ECG characteristic
- Rate: difficult to ascertain, fibrillation waves are seen at a rate in excess of 300/min
- Rhythm: irregular, uncoordinated, chaotic
- P waves: may or may not be present, but anyway are unrecognizable
- P–R interval: absent
- QRS complex: absent. The ectopic foci result in waves of fibrillation of varying amplitude and shape. The waves are known as coarse or fine depending upon amplitude.

Clinical significance
May have the same causes as the other ventricular dysrhythmias.
Ventricular fibrillation will result in a total loss of cardiac output, and cause cardiac arrest.

Treatment
Cardiac arrest, page 52.

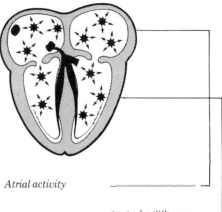

Figure 22(a). Ventricular fibrillation

Atrial activity

Ventricular activity

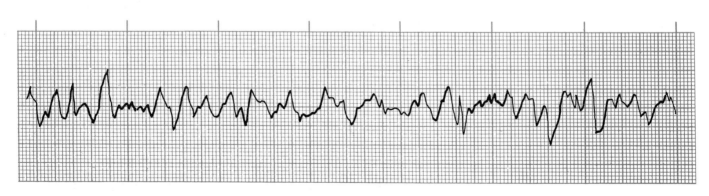

Figure 22(b). Ventricular fibrillation (coarse → fine)

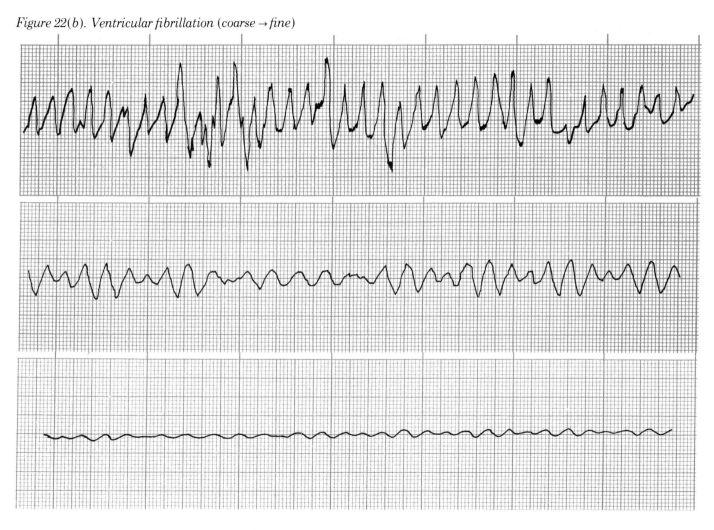

Ventricular standstill

Description
Total absence of ventricular activity. Atrial activity only is seen (figure 23).

ECG characteristic
- Rate: ventricular — nil. Atrial rate may be normal
- Rhythm: absent
- P waves: normal
- P–R interval: not identifiable
- QRS complex: absent

Clinical significance
Results in an absence of cardiac output, that is cardiac arrest.

Treatment
Cardiac arrest, page 52.

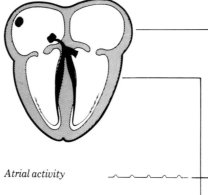

Figure 23. Ventricular standstill

Atrial activity

No ventricular activity

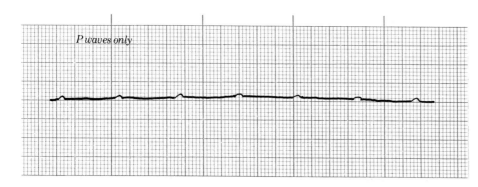

P waves only

Ventricular flutter

This term may be used to describe a form of ventricular fibrillation which is seen as a series of large wave-like oscillations (figure 24).

Figure 24

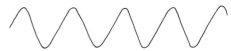

Asystole

There is a total absence of myocardial activity resulting in a loss of cardiac output. Occasionally some bizarre-looking movement may be noted on the trace, at an extremely slow rate, often called *post-mortem artefact* or *dying heart syndrome* (figure 25). Otherwise, all that can be seen is basically the isoelectric line on the monitor with some slight movement; rarely is it a perfectly straight line. For treatment see section on cardiac arrest, page 52.

Figure 25

Heart block

When a conduction defect exists impulses may be delayed in their passage through the heart or even be totally prevented from passing to the ventricles. This is called heart block and it can be divided into several types.

First-degree heart block

Description
Here the impulse originates as normal in the S-A node but the conduction through the A-V node is slowed beyond normal limits, resulting in a longer than normal P–R interval. The rest of the complex is normal (figure 26).

ECG characteristic
- Rate: normal
- Rhythm: regular
- P waves: normal
- P–R interval: greater than 0.2 sec
- QRS complex: normal

Clinical significance
It may be caused by damage to the A-V node (as a result of organic heart disease), increased parasympathetic tone on the A-V node, hypoxia or overdose of some drugs, such as digoxin. If the rate is normal there may be no effect on the patient. The rhythm need only be noted because of an abnormally slow rate.

Treatment
No treatment is indicated if the rate is normal (if excessively slow it may be treated as sinus bradycardia, page 8). If, however, it is associated with organic heart disease (myocardial infarction, for example) the patient should be observed as the rhythm may progress to second- or third-degree heart block.

Figure 26. First-degree heart block

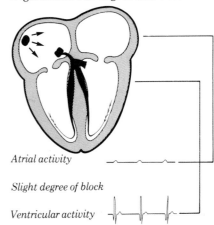

Atrial activity

Slight degree of block

Ventricular activity

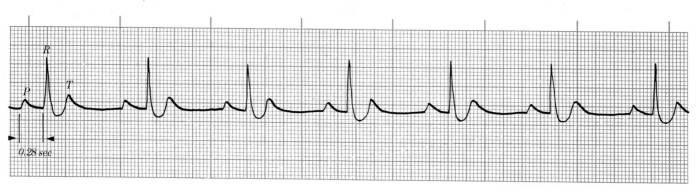

Second-degree heart block

This is further subdivided into:
(1) Mobitz type I (or Wenckebach phenomenon)
(2) Mobitz type II

Mobitz type I (Wenckebach phenomenon)

Description
The impulse originates in the S-A node as normal, but the conduction through the A-V node is abnormal. The impulse is delayed slightly longer each time it passes through the A-V node. This results in an increasing P–R interval until eventually one impulse from the S-A node is completely blocked while the impulse following is allowed to pass through the A-V node at a more normal interval. This is seen on the ECG as an increasing P–R interval until a P wave is seen that is not followed by a QRS complex. This is usually seen as a cycle with one more P wave in the cycle than QRS complexes (although the number of complexes in each cycle may occasionally vary) (figure 27).

ECG characteristic
■ Rate: normal or slow
■ Rhythm: P waves regular; QRS complexes irregular
■ P waves: normal
■ P–R interval: increasing in length in each cycle. May be normal at the beginning of the cycle.
■ QRS complex: normal

Clinical significance
May be caused for the same reasons as first-degree heart block. If the rate is normal there may be little or no effect on the patient. If the rate is excessively slow cardiac output may deteriorate, resulting in the signs and symptoms of low cardiac output.

Treatment
If the cardiac output is normal, no treatment is required. Although the rhythm does carry the risk of deterioration to complete heart block. If the patient does show the signs and symptoms of a reduced cardiac output, in other words a drop in blood pressure, peripheral vasoconstriction, poor tissue perfusion, confusion and even unconsciousness, he will require oxygen to relieve the hypoxia. Atropine sulphate may be of help as it increases the rate at the S-A node and therefore the ventricular rate.

An isoprenaline infusion or pacemaker insertion may be required if the patient's cardiac output is very low.

Figure 27. Mobitz type I (Wenckebach phenomenon)

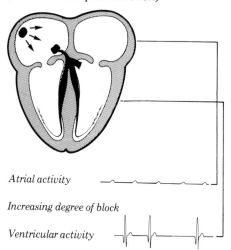

Atrial activity

Increasing degree of block

Ventricular activity

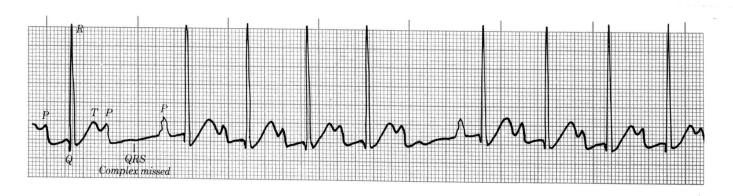

Mobitz type II

Description
Very similar to Mobitz type I, the difference being that the A-V node blocks a regular number of impulses allowing every second, third or fourth, etc. impulse through to stimulate the ventricles. The rate of block is usually regular, but may be irregular. The individual rhythm may be described as a 2 : 1, 3 : 1, 4 : 1, etc. block depending upon how many P waves are noted prior to each QRS complex (figure 28).

ECG characteristic
- Rate: normal or slow
- Rhythm: P waves regular; QRS complexes regular (occasionally irregular)
- P waves: normal
- P–R interval: When seen it may be normal or prolonged but is constant. There may be two, three or more P waves prior to each QRS complex.
- QRS complex: normal or occasionally widened

Clinical significance
The same as Mobitz type I.

Treatment
As for Mobitz type I.

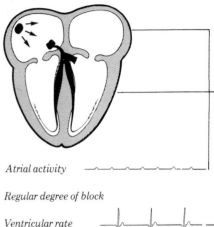

Figure 28. Mobitz type II

Atrial activity

Regular degree of block

Ventricular rate

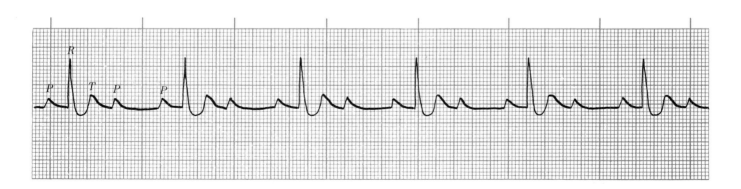

Third-degree heart block

This is also known as complete heart block or complete atrioventricular dissociation.

Description
The A-V node does not conduct any impulses and therefore the atria and ventricles beat completely independently of each other. The S-A node continues to pace the atria but because the impulses are not conducted through the A-V node an ectopic focus in the ventricles takes over the control of the ventricles. If the ectopic focus is high up in the ventricles near the bundle of His the QRS complexes may appear quite normal. If the ectopic focus is low in the ventricles the QRS complex may appear wide and bizarre. The P waves and QRS complexes have no relationship to each other, and the P waves are often lost in the QRS complexes. Occasionally a P wave may be seen prior to the QRS complex, but this is purely a coincidence, and the two have no relationship to each other, and are completely dissociated (figure 29).

ECG characteristic
- Rate: atrial rate may be normal; ventricular rate may be 20–50 bpm
- Rhythm: atria regular; ventricles usually regular
- P waves: normal, but may not be seen as they may be buried in the QRS complexes
- P–R interval: absent
- QRS complex: abnormal, the width and shape may vary depending upon exact focus

Clinical significance
The rhythm may be caused by damage to the A-V node, bundle of His or bundle branches (as in ischaemic heart disease or trauma) or increased parasympathetic tone. The ventricular rate is usually low with its associated lowering of cardiac output. The patient, therefore, will show the signs and symptoms of the lowered cardiac output; because of the slow rate ventricular dysrhythmias may appear, and there is also the risk of deterioration to ventricular standstill.

Treatment
If the rate is sufficient to maintain cardiac output little treatment may be required.

If the patient shows the signs and symptoms of the lowered cardiac output supportive therapy, such as oxygen therapy or entonox will be required. An isoprenaline infusion may also be required — 4 mg of isoprenaline is added to 1000 ml of 5% dextrose and run through a Metriset, initially at 15 ml/h (15 drops/min). The rate may be altered depending upon the ventricular response.

A pacemaker may also be inserted, temporary for the emergency and, if necessary a permanent pacemaker later.

Figure 29. Third-degree heart block (complete heart block)

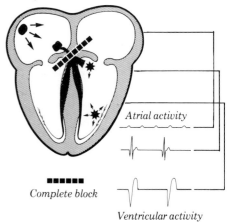

Atrial activity

Complete block

Ventricular activity

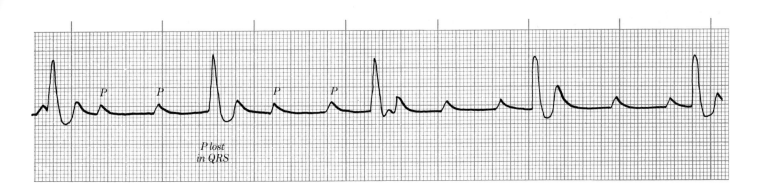

P   *P*   *P*   *P*

P lost
in QRS

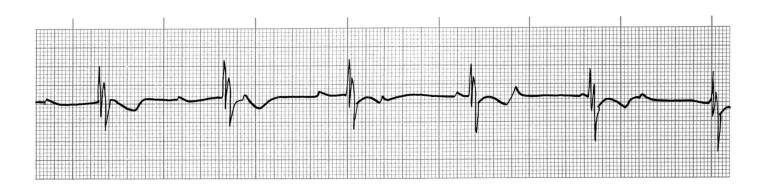

Stokes–Adams attack

Description
The underlying rhythm may be regular and relatively normal, or there may be some degree of heart block. There is a sudden loss of cardiac output resulting in the associated signs and symptoms. The rhythm causing this is often ventricular standstill, but may occasionally be ventricular fibrillation or asystole.

The rhythm may revert spontaneously or may need active treatment to revert to a more normal rhythm (figure 30).

ECG characteristic
- Rate: during attack — nil
- Rhythm: may or may not be normal, during attack will be absent.
- P waves: may or may not be present
- P–R interval: absent
- QRS complex: absent during the attack

Clinical significance
The dysrhythmia may be caused by any of the reasons which may cause heart block.

The sudden total loss of cardiac output

produces a dizzy episode (within 5 sec), loss of consciousness (after 10 sec), fits (after 15 sec) and apparent death after 30 sec. If the patient does not revert spontaneously death will ensue unless he is resuscitated.

Occasionally if the patient is upright when the Stokes–Adams attack occurs the jolt as he hits the ground may revert the dysrhythmia and he may appear to have just fainted.

Treatment
If the patient reverts spontaneously, general observation may be all that is required (including monitor observation). Oxygen therapy may be necessary if the patient is hypoxic. If he does not revert spontaneously he will show the signs and symptoms of cardiac arrest. (For treatment see section on cardiac arrest, page 52).

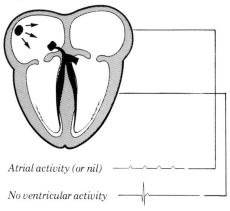

Figure 30. Stokes–Adams attack

Atrial activity (or nil)

No ventricular activity

May revert spontaneously

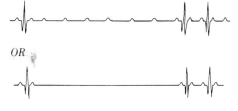

OR

OR

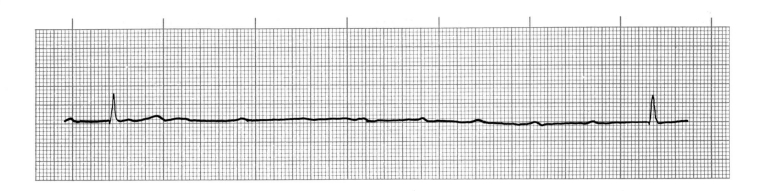

47

Paced beats

Description
Because the underlying rhythm is abnormal and very slow an electrical pacemaker is used to increase the ventricular rate. The end of the pacing catheter is lodged in the apex of the right ventricle. The P waves and paced beats may or may not appear dissociated from each other. Though the QRS complex seen appears wide and bizarre it results in a good ventricular output (figure 31).

An upright faint line may be noted at the start of the QRS complex; this is the pacing artefact caused by the pacing stimulus.

ECG characteristic
- Rate: ventricular rate normal (70–80 bpm)
- Rhythm: regular
- P waves: may or may not be noted
- P–R interval: absent
- QRS complex: wide and bizarre

Clinical significance
The treatment of a dysrhythmia (complete heart block) therefore will result in an improvement in the patient's condition, in other words, a normal heart rate and satisfactory cardiac output.

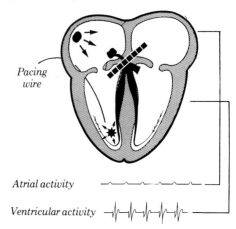

Figure 31. Paced beats (internal pacemaker)

Pacing wire

Atrial activity

Ventricular activity

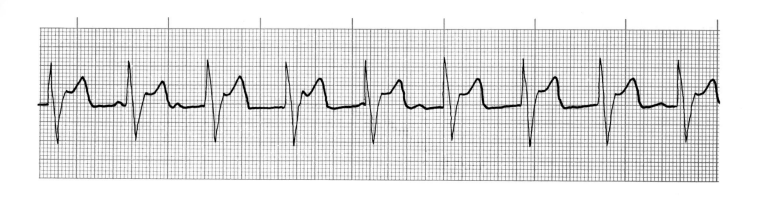

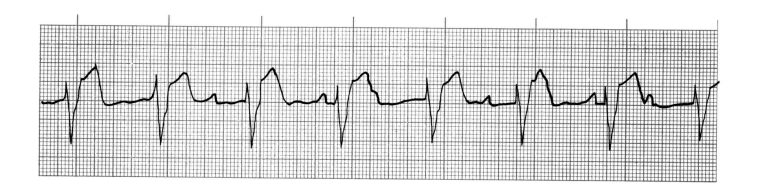

49

Bundle branch block

This occurs when there is damage to one of the branches of the bundle of His, and results in an abnormal conduction of the impulse through the bundle branches. This may be seen on the QRS complex as a notch, the position of the notch varying according to the position of the block. A 12-lead ECG is needed to diagnose whether right or left bundle branch block is present.

The bundle branch block may be of little significance, or may be the precursor of a total block at the bundle of His.

It is important to note on the monitor that this is recognized as an addition on an underlying rhythm. For example, a notch on the QRS complex but no P wave would be suggestive of a mid-nodal rhythm, but if the notch is seen and a P wave is noted prior to the complex then a bundle branch block may be seen (figure 32).

Figure 32.

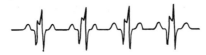

Signs of myocardial ischaemia, injury and infarction

It is important first to remember that to diagnose accurately myocardial ischaemia, injury or infarction on the ECG, a 12-lead ECG must be recorded. Occasionally the signs may be seen on a monitoring lead, but as these signs can only be *suggestive* of ischaemia, injury or infarction they are not conclusive or diagnostic.

If an area of the myocardium is infarcted the muscle cells cannot be polarized or depolarized, so if an electrode is placed over this area it will only pick up the electrical activity opposite (as if looking through a 'window').

If an area of myocardium is only ischaemic or injured then abnormalities of the T wave and S–T segment may be seen on an electrode placed over the ischaemic or injured area.

Ischaemia: May be seen as an inverted T wave, in a patient who complains of angina (ischaemic heart disease), or it may be seen in a routine examination.

Injury: This is seen as a raised S–T segment, usually the higher the S–T segment the greater the degree of injury.

Infarction: This is seen as a deep Q wave (greater than a third the depth of the total height/depth of the QRS complex), in combination with the signs of ischaemia and injury.

Around an area of infarction is an area of injury which in turn is surrounded by an area of ischaemia (see figure 33).

If the electrode used is placed on the opposite side of the infarction, injury or ischaemia, the opposite or reciprocal effect will be seen on the ECG.

Figure 33. Signs of myocardial ischaemia, injury and infarction on the ECG

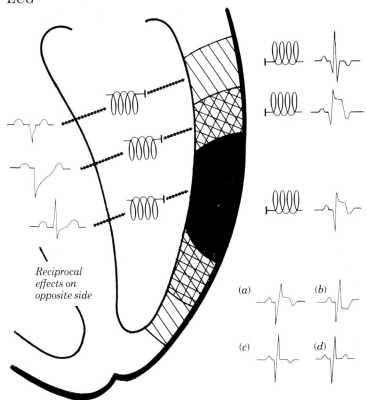

Reciprocal effects on opposite side

Ischaemia results in a depressed T wave due to altered repolarization

Myocardial injury results in elevation of the S–T segment

Death of myocardium (infarction) results in a deep Q wave. (picks up depolarization from the opposite wall)

During recovery the S–T segment often becomes depressed, then returns to normal. The T wave also returns to normal but the Q wave remains.

 Area of ischaemia   Area of injury   Area of infarction

Cardiac arrest

For a fuller treatment of this topic, see J. Gardiner, *Cardiac Arrest — What Do You Do?* (Stanley Thornes Publishers, 1986)

By definition, cardiac arrest is a failure of the heart to maintain an adequate cerebral circulation in the absence of a causative or irreversible disease. This tells us that cardiac arrest is a potentially reversible situation while death, of course, is not.

Although there may be many causes of cardiac arrest, both the effect on the patient and the treatment are the same.

Effect on the patient

If the circulation stops, and therefore the blood flow to the brain ceases, the partial pressure of oxygen (PO_2) in the cerebral vessels will drop to 20 mmHg within 10 sec causing loss of consciousness. The cerebral PO_2 drops to zero within approximately 1 min causing respiration to cease. Within minutes of this occurrence there is irreversible brain damage. As the blood flow to the tissues has ceased there is a general tissue hypoxia and a build-up of waste products, as they cannot be removed. This leads to several effects, of which the most important is the lactic acidosis produced by the anaerobic respiration. All these effects lead to a number of signs that can be used to diagnose cardiac arrest. But there are two main signs that will always be present and these two alone are all that are required to diagnose cardiac arrest.

Diagnosis

The two primary signs that are required are:
(1) unconsciousness,
(2) loss of arterial pulses (carotid, femoral).

If these signs are present the patient is in a state of cardiac arrest. Other signs develop as the general tissue and cerebral hypoxia increase, and there is irreversible brain damage.

Cerebral signs
Respiration ceases (similarly respiratory arrest leads to cardiac arrest if untreated); pupils dilate and become unresponsive.

General signs
There is pallor or greyness (other colours may be seen depending upon cause of arrest, such as the cherry red colour of carbon monoxide poisoning); cyanosis, central and/or peripheral; cold, clammy skin.

Treatment

The initial management consists of three main areas:

(1) Airway: must be cleared,
(2) Breathing: initiate expired air resuscitation,
(3) Circulation: imitate with external chest compression.

Airway
This may be cleared and maintained solely by the use of suction and good position. The aid of either an oropharyngeal airway, or later after the initial oxygenation (if required) endotracheal intubation may be necessary.

Breathing
If the patient only has a cardiac arrest and is still breathing himself, assisted ventilation may not be required. However by the time resuscitation is implemented the patient often has had a respiratory arrest.

Initial ventilation may be by expired air resuscitation until a bag and mask are available. The patient should be ventilated until adequately oxygenated (with added oxygen if available), and if necessary intubated to aid airway care during ventilation.

Circulation
If the patient is seen to 'collapse', implementation of the precordial 'thump' may be useful. If the patient has had a Stokes–Adams attack this may be sufficient to revert him. If cardiac arrest continues external chest compression (ECC) must be implemented.

Both assisted ventilation and ECC must be continued throughout resuscitation attempts. The efficiency of ECC can be checked by feeling for a carotid or femoral pulse, and this should be felt with each compression. If ventilation and ECC are satisfactorily continued the patient's colour should improve and dilated pupils constrict. After the initial management, at a convenient time an ECG monitor should be attached to the patient by the standard limb leads, to assess the rhythm. This can be quite variable and could look relatively normal, but it usually includes ventricular fibrillation, ventricular standstill or asystole. While the monitor is observed there must be a pause in ECC as this will cause an artefact on the monitor. The only other times that there is a pause in ECC, or it is stopped, is during defibrillation, on recovery of the patient, or when resuscitation is abandoned.

Defibrillation
If the patient is seen to be in coarse ventricular fibrillation (VF), defibrillation is required as soon as possible. The technique of charging varies slightly with different types of defibrillator, but the use and dangers are the same with each.

The patient and defibrillator paddles must be adequately jelled with electrode jelly to minimize the risk of burns to the patient. The electrode jelly must be in two distinctly separate areas; if the two connect the current may arc across the chest and burn the patient (alternatively there are squares of 'solid' gel available which ensure that an adequate area of the patient's chest is covered). The paddles should be applied firmly to the patient's chest, one slightly to the right of the sternum at the level of the 2nd to 4th ribs, and the second just below the apex of the heart.

The monitor should be checked immediately prior to defibrillation to ensure that the patient has not reverted spontaneously.

During defibrillation ensure that no one is touching the patient, or anything that the patient is touching; especially bystanders. The shock may convert them to ventricular fibrillation. Resuscitation may need to be recommenced immediately after defibrillation if there is no cardiac output, followed by a repeat defibrillation if the patient is still in VF.

To defibrillate the adult 200 Joules (J) are used increasing to 360 J. A child will require 2 J/kg body weight, increasing if necessary to 4 J/kg.

If a patient is in ventricular fibrillation he needs to be defibrillated, and the sooner it is done the better his chance of recovery.

Note: The legs can be raised slightly (approximately 30°) to aid the venous return to the heart. The head must not be lowered as high cerebral venous pressure may lead to cerebral oedema and increased cerebral hypoxia.

Failure of asystole to revert to ventricular fibrillation, or persistent ventricular fibrillation, may be indicative of severe myocardial damage.

Persistent pupil dilation, despite adequate resuscitation, may indicate irreversible cerebral damage.

Figure 34. Arrhythmias that may be seen prior to or during a cardiac arrest

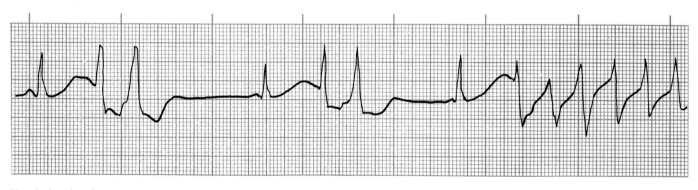

Ventricular trigeminy ⟶ Ventricular tachycardia

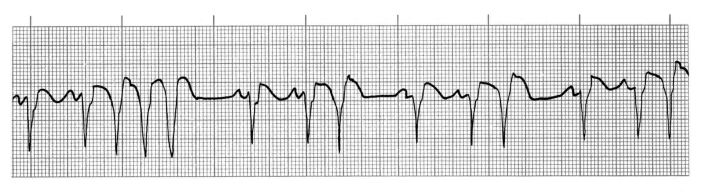

*Sinus rhythm with frequent
ventricular ectopics*

*Ventricular
tachycardia*

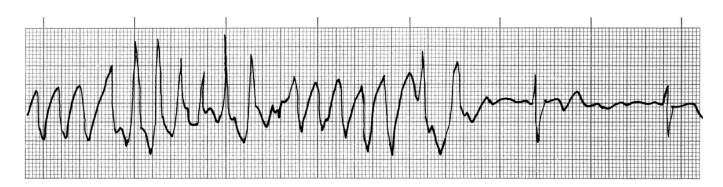

*Spontaneous reversion of ventricular fibrillation
to a more normal rhythm.*

Secondary treatment of cardiac arrest

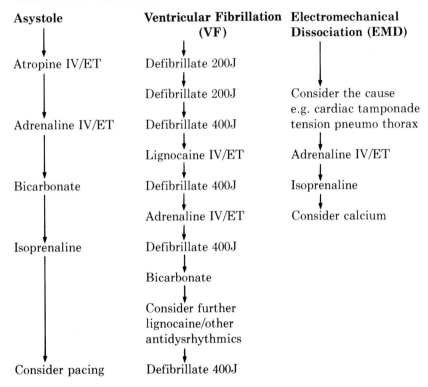

Asystole	Ventricular Fibrillation (VF)	Electromechanical Dissociation (EMD)
↓	↓	↓
Atropine IV/ET	Defibrillate 200J	
↓	↓	
	Defibrillate 200J	Consider the cause
	↓	e.g. cardiac tamponade
Adrenaline IV/ET	Defibrillate 400J	tension pneumo thorax
↓	↓	↓
	Lignocaine IV/ET	Adrenaline IV/ET
	↓	↓
Bicarbonate	Defibrillate 400J	Isoprenaline
↓	↓	↓
	Adrenaline IV/ET	Consider calcium
↓	↓	
Isoprenaline	Defibrillate 400J	
↓	↓	
	Bicarbonate	
	↓	
	Consider further lignocaine/other antidysrhythmics	
↓	↓	
Consider pacing	Defibrillate 400J	

IV/ET may be given intravenously or via the endotracheal tube.
All other drugs given intravenously.

(the above guidelines follow the recommendations of © The Resuscitation Council (UK))

Drugs used in the management of cardiac arrest

Adrenaline
1 mg IV (2 mg via ET tube).
Used in the management of Asystole, Electrochemical dissociation and Ventricular Fibrillation resistant to defibrillation.

Atropine
2 mg IV (4 mg via ET tube).
May follow adrenaline in the management of asystole.

Lignocaine
100 mg IV (200 mg via ET tube).
May follow adrenaline in the management of Ventricular Fibrillation resistant to defibrillation.

During the management of prolonged cardiac arrest Sodium Bicarbonate may be considered after the estimation of arterial blood gases.

Success or ?

If resuscitation is successful the patient's colour should improve, and pupils constrict. If the cardiac output returns a pulse will be felt, and if the hypoxia has been relieved respiratory effort may return and the patient may gradually recover consciousness.

If the patient fails to respond to resuscitation, in other words, there is still no pulse and no respiration, the colour is poor, and pupils are fixed and dilated, continue ventilation and ECC until a decision to abandon resuscitation is made.

Aftercare

When the patient is recovering, the following steps should be taken.

(1) Maintain care of the airway with assisted ventilation if required.
(2) Observe consciousness level, heart rate, respirations, monitor etc.
(3) Give oxygen therapy — 28% ventimask until blood gases are assessed.
(4) If the period of hypoxia has led to the onset of cerebral oedema, give *Dexamethasone* 4–12 mg i.v., which can be followed by 10% *mannitol* later if necessary.
(5) Check for injuries incurred during resuscitation or at the initial collapse and treat as necessary. (For example, fractured ribs, flail segment, pneumothorax, head injury, etc.). Also assess for the presence of left ventricular failure, etc.
(6) Discover why the patient had a cardiac arrest. Observe him — he may have it again!
(7) If the patient is conscious and distressed reassure him. If necessary give Valium (2.5–5 mg i.v.), with care as this may cause the blood pressure to drop.

Index